Understanding and Overcoming Hernias:

A Patient's Guide

Dr. James W. Mosley

This book aims to be a comprehensive guide, providing practical information, emotional support, and empowering patients to actively manage their hernia journey.

DEDICATION

This book is dedicated to my family and to everyone going through hernia.

TABLE OF CONTENTS

UNDERSTANDING AND OVERCOMING HERNIAS

Chapter 1: Unveiling Hernias

Exploring the anatomy of hernias

In our quest to understand and overcome hernias, it is essential to embark on a journey into the intricate world of human anatomy. A hernia, in its simplest terms, occurs when an internal organ or tissue pushes through a weakened spot in the surrounding muscle or connective tissue. This breach can lead to a visible bulge or lump, often causing discomfort or pain. To comprehend this phenomenon, let's delve into the fundamental aspects of hernia anatomy.

At the heart of our exploration lies the understanding that muscles and connective tissues form the structural framework of our bodies. They work seamlessly together to maintain the integrity of our various organs. However, vulnerabilities can emerge over time, giving rise to potential weak points. Hernias typically exploit these weakened areas.

The abdominal region, being a focal point for hernias, demands particular attention. Within this expanse, we find a network of muscles and tissues responsible for supporting organs such as the intestines. It is in this intricate tapestry that hernias find their canvas.

Visualizing the anatomy of hernias extends beyond textbook descriptions. It necessitates an exploration of the dynamics that govern the relationship between muscles, tissues, and organs. This intricate dance is susceptible to disruptions, and hernias represent a choreography gone awry.

For patients grappling with the reality of a hernia, this understanding becomes a compass guiding them through the complexities of their condition. It empowers them to decipher medical jargon, engage in informed discussions with healthcare professionals, and actively participate in decisions regarding their care.

In essence, our exploration of hernia anatomy unveils a narrative of vulnerability and resilience within the human body. It is a narrative that beckons us to appreciate the delicate balance between strength and susceptibility, and in doing so, enables us to navigate the path toward healing and recovery.

Anatomy of Hernias: A Deeper Look

The abdominal wall plays a pivotal role in supporting and protecting internal organs. Comprising layers of muscles, connective tissue, and fascia, it acts as a robust barrier. However, weaknesses or openings in this wall can lead to the development of hernias.

1. Layers of the Abdominal Wall:

External Oblique Muscle: This is the outermost muscle layer of the abdominal wall, providing strength and stability.

Internal Oblique Muscle: Situated beneath the external oblique, it contributes to the overall integrity of the abdominal wall.

Transversus Abdominis Muscle: The deepest muscle layer, playing a key role in maintaining abdominal pressure.

2. Fascia and Connective Tissue:

Linea Alba: Running vertically along the midline of the abdomen, it is a tough band of connective tissue that connects the muscles on either side.

Inguinal Ligament: Located in the groin, it provides support to the abdominal wall.

3. Potential Weak Points:

Inguinal Canal: An area where blood vessels and structures like the spermatic cord pass through. Weaknesses in this region can lead to inguinal hernias.

Femoral Canal: Another potential site for hernias, located just below the inguinal ligament.

Factors like genetics, aging, and increased abdominal pressure contribute to the vulnerabilities in these areas, paving the way for hernia formation. By unraveling the intricacies of abdominal anatomy, individuals can better appreciate the mechanisms behind hernias and make informed decisions about prevention and treatment.

Types of hernias and their common locations

Let's explore the various types of hernias and their common locations in more detail:

1. Inguinal Hernias:
   Common Location: In the inguinal canal, situated in the groin. This is the most

prevalent type of hernia and is more common in men.

Description: Inguinal hernias can be further classified as direct or indirect. Direct hernias protrude through weakened areas In the abdominal wall, while indirect hernias involve the inguinal canal.

2. Femoral Hernias:

Common Location: Below the inguinal ligament, in the femoral canal. More common in women.

Description: These hernias occur when abdominal contents, such as a part of the intestine, protrude through the femoral canal, creating a bulge in the upper thigh.

3. Hiatal Hernias:

Common Location: At the opening in the diaphragm where the esophagus passes through (hiatus). This type is located in the upper part of the stomach.

Description: Hiatal hernias result in a portion of the stomach sliding into the chest through the diaphragmatic opening, leading to symptoms like acid reflux.

4. Umbilical Hernias:
   Common Location: Near the navel (umbilicus).
   Description: Often seen in infants, umbilical hernias occur when a small part of the intestine protrudes through the abdominal muscles near the belly button. While common in babies, they can persist or develop in adults.

5. Incisional Hernias:
   Common Location: Develop at the site of a previous surgical incision or scar.
   Description: Incisional hernias occur when tissue or organs protrude through a weakened area in the abdominal wall created by a previous surgical procedure.

6. Epigastric Hernias:
   Common Location: Between the breastbone (sternum) and the navel (umbilicus).

Description: These hernias involve fatty tissue pushing through a weakened area in the upper abdominal wall. They may not always cause noticeable bulges but can lead to discomfort.

Understanding the specific characteristics and locations of each type of hernia is crucial for accurate diagnosis and appropriate treatment. While some hernias may be asymptomatic, others can cause pain, discomfort, or complications, emphasizing the importance of timely medical attention. Each type of hernia requires a tailored approach for effective management and, in some cases, surgical intervention to repair the weakened abdominal wall.

Recognizing early symptoms and signs

Recognizing the early symptoms and signs of hernias is pivotal for individuals to seek timely medical attention and initiate appropriate management. While hernias may initially be asymptomatic, early detection can prevent complications and facilitate more effective treatment.

The most common manifestation of a hernia is a noticeable bulge or lump in the affected area. In inguinal hernias, for example, this bulge often appears in the groin and may become more pronounced when standing, coughing, or lifting heavy objects. In femoral hernias, the bulge typically presents in the upper thigh and can be accompanied by a feeling of pressure or discomfort. Hiatal hernias may cause symptoms like heartburn, regurgitation, and difficulty swallowing due to stomach acid moving into the esophagus.

Pain or discomfort is another early indicator of hernias. Individuals may experience a dull ache or sharp pain at the site of the bulge, especially during activities that increase abdominal pressure. In some cases, the pain may be intermittent, making it crucial for individuals to pay attention to any unusual sensations in the abdominal region.

Changes in bowel habits can also be indicative of certain hernias. Constipation, bloating, or difficulty passing gas may occur due to the protrusion of abdominal contents impacting normal digestive processes. For hiatal hernias, symptoms may extend beyond the abdominal region, with individuals reporting chest pain, belching, and a sensation of fullness after meals.

It's essential to recognize that hernias can be more than physical bulges or discomfort. Persistent feelings of fatigue or weakness may signal the presence of an underlying hernia, as the body expends extra energy to compensate for the strain on the abdominal wall. Additionally, some individuals may experience a dragging sensation or heaviness in the affected area.

While these signs may seem subtle initially, it's crucial not to dismiss them, as hernias have the potential to worsen over time. Regular self examinations, especially in high risk individuals or those with a family history of hernias, can aid in the early detection of any unusual changes in the abdominal region.

In conclusion, recognizing the early symptoms and signs of hernias involves a combination of physical awareness and vigilance. Being attuned to changes in the abdominal region, including the appearance of a bulge, sensations of pain or discomfort, and alterations in bowel habits, empowers individuals to take proactive steps toward seeking medical advice. Early intervention can significantly impact the management of hernias, potentially preventing complications and facilitating a smoother path to recovery.

Chapter 2: Navigating Symptoms

In-depth discussion on symptoms for various hernia types

An in-depth exploration of the symptoms associated with various types of hernias is crucial for individuals to recognize potential signs and seek timely medical evaluation. The diverse nature of hernias means that symptoms can manifest differently depending on the location and type of hernia.

Inguinal Hernias:
Inguinal hernias, being the most common type, often present with a noticeable bulge or lump in the groin area. This bulge may become more prominent when standing, coughing, or lifting heavy objects. In addition to the physical protrusion, individuals may experience discomfort, pain, or a dragging sensation. It's not uncommon for inguinal hernias to cause a

feeling of fullness or pressure in the affected region.

Femoral Hernias:
Femoral hernias typically manifest as a bulge in the upper thigh, below the inguinal ligament. Individuals may notice a tender lump in this area, accompanied by discomfort or a feeling of heaviness. Due to their location, femoral hernias can be prone to complications, making it imperative to identify and address symptoms promptly.

Hiatal Hernias:
The symptoms of hiatal hernias often extend beyond the abdominal region. Heartburn, regurgitation, and difficulty swallowing are common indicators. Individuals may experience chest pain or discomfort, resembling symptoms of acid reflux. Hiatal hernias can also cause bloating, belching, and a feeling of fullness, especially after meals.

Umbilical Hernias:

Umbilical hernias, prevalent in infants and sometimes persisting into adulthood, are characterized by a bulge near the navel. While they may be asymptomatic, some individuals may notice tenderness or aching at the site of the hernia. In infants, crying or increased abdominal pressure during activities like crying or coughing can accentuate the bulge.

Incisional Hernias:
Developing at the site of a previous surgical incision or scar, incisional hernias may not always present with a visible bulge. Instead, individuals may experience pain or discomfort around the scar area. Activities that increase intraabdominal pressure, such as lifting heavy objects, can exacerbate these symptoms.

Understanding the nuances of symptoms associated with each hernia type is instrumental in early detection and appropriate medical intervention. While some hernias may be asymptomatic, others can cause persistent discomfort or lead to complications if left untreated. As such, individuals should remain vigilant, promptly consult healthcare professionals when experiencing symptoms, and undergo thorough assessments to determine the best course of action for their specific hernia type. Early diagnosis and intervention can significantly contribute to successful treatment outcomes and improved quality of life.

Understanding when to seek medical attention

Understanding when to seek medical attention for hernias is paramount, as early intervention can prevent complications and improve treatment outcomes. While some hernias may be asymptomatic or cause mild discomfort, certain signs necessitate prompt evaluation by healthcare professionals.

Persistent Pain or Discomfort: Persistent pain or discomfort in the abdominal region, especially around a noticeable bulge, should not be ignored. While occasional discomfort may not raise immediate concern, ongoing or increasing pain may indicate complications such as strangulation or obstruction. Seeking medical attention promptly allows healthcare providers to assess the severity of the situation and recommend appropriate interventions.

Changes in Appearance or Size of the Bulge: If there is a hernia present, any noticeable changes in its appearance or size warrant medical evaluation. An increase in size may indicate the progression of the hernia or the development of complications. Conversely, sudden changes, such as a bulge becoming firm or tender, could signify a more urgent situation, requiring immediate medical attention to prevent potential complications like bowel obstruction.

Difficulty with Bowel Movements or Blood Flow:
Hernias can sometimes impact normal bowel function. Symptoms such as difficulty passing stool, persistent constipation, or the presence of blood in the stool necessitate prompt medical assessment. These signs could indicate complications such as bowel obstruction or compromised blood flow, both of which require immediate attention to prevent serious consequences.

Associated Symptoms in Hiatal Hernias:
For hiatal hernias, symptoms extending beyond the abdominal region, such as chest pain, difficulty swallowing, or persistent heartburn, should prompt a medical consultation. These symptoms may indicate complications related to the displacement of the stomach into the chest cavity, and

addressing them early can prevent further discomfort and potential complications.

Unexplained Fatigue or Weakness:
General feelings of fatigue or weakness that cannot be attributed to other factors may be associated with hernias. The body may exert additional energy to compensate for the strain caused by the hernia. Identifying and addressing these systemic symptoms early can aid in preventing further complications and promoting overall wellbeing.

Inability to Reduce or Push the Hernia Back In:
Individuals who notice a hernia and are unable to push it back in, or reduce it, should seek immediate medical attention. This inability to reduce the hernia may indicate complications such as incarceration or strangulation, which require urgent medical intervention.

In summary, recognizing when to seek medical attention for hernias involves attentiveness to changes in symptoms, prompt evaluation of persistent pain or discomfort, and awareness of signs that may indicate complications. Timely medical consultation allows healthcare professionals to conduct thorough assessments, determine the appropriate course of action, and intervene early to manage hernias effectively. Being proactive in seeking medical attention empowers individuals to address hernias in their early stages, minimizing the risk of complications and promoting optimal outcomes in treatment and recovery.

Illustrative patient stories to connect with readers

Patient Story 1: Emily's Journey to Recovery

Meet Emily, a vibrant 35yearold who discovered an inguinal hernia during a routine workout. At first, she dismissed the discomfort as muscle strain, but as a visible bulge appeared, Emily decided to consult her doctor. The diagnosis revealed an inguinal hernia. Emily opted for surgical repair and, after a thorough recovery process, she's back to her active lifestyle, emphasizing the importance of early detection and seeking medical attention.

Patient Story 2: Carlos and His Umbilical Hernia

Carlos, a father of two, noticed a small bulge near his belly button that grew over time. Concerned about the impact on his family life, he consulted a healthcare professional who diagnosed an umbilical hernia. Despite initial worries, Carlos underwent a successful surgical procedure, and his recovery allowed him to fully engage in family activities again. His story highlights the emotional journey of coping with a hernia and the positive impact of timely intervention.

Patient Story 3: Sarah's Triumph Over Hiatal Hernia Challenges

Sarah, a 40yearold professional, experienced persistent heartburn and difficulty swallowing, affecting her work and personal life. After consulting with her healthcare team, she was diagnosed with a hiatal hernia. Sarah opted for a comprehensive treatment plan, combining lifestyle changes and medication. Through perseverance and support, Sarah regained control over her symptoms, emphasizing that managing hiatal hernias often involves a holistic approach and patient dedication.

Patient Story 4: Tom's Incisional Hernia Recovery

Tom, in his mid50s, developed an incisional hernia following abdominal surgery. Faced with discomfort and concern about a recurrence, he consulted his surgeon for guidance. Tom's experience underscores the importance of communication between patients and healthcare providers. Following a successful hernia repair, Tom actively participates in support groups, sharing insights on the significance of postsurgical care and ongoing wellbeing.

Chapter 3: Treatment Options

Surgical and nonsurgical approaches

Surgical Approaches:

Herniorrhaphy:
One of the most common surgical procedures for hernias is herniorrhaphy. In this approach, the surgeon makes an incision over the hernia site, pushes the protruding tissue back into place, and repairs the weakened abdominal wall using stitches or synthetic mesh. This method is effective for various hernia types, including inguinal, femoral, and incisional hernias.

Laparoscopic Hernia Repair:
Laparoscopic or minimally invasive surgery involves smaller incisions and the use of a tiny camera (laparoscope) to guide the surgeon. Through these small incisions, the hernia is repaired with the assistance of specialized instruments. Laparoscopic procedures often result in shorter recovery

times, reduced pain, and less scarring compared to traditional open surgery.

Robotic-Assisted Hernia Repair:
Robotic-assisted surgery combines advanced robotic technology with a surgeon's expertise. The surgeon controls robotic arms to perform the operation through small incisions. This approach offers enhanced precision and maneuverability, particularly beneficial in complex or recurrent hernia cases.

Non-surgical Approaches:

Watchful Waiting:
In certain cases, especially when hernias are small and asymptomatic, a watchful waiting approach may be recommended. Regular monitoring, lifestyle adjustments, and close communication with healthcare professionals help manage the condition without immediate surgical intervention.

Supportive Garments:

Compression garments, such as hernia belts or trusses, provide external support to the weakened abdominal area. While these do not cure hernias, they can alleviate symptoms and offer temporary relief. Healthcare professionals may recommend their use before or after surgery or in cases where surgery is not an immediate option.

Lifestyle Modifications:
Addressing risk factors through lifestyle changes can be crucial. This includes maintaining a healthy weight, avoiding activities that strain the abdominal muscles, and managing conditions like chronic coughing or constipation. These modifications aim to reduce the likelihood of hernia development or recurrence.

Physical Therapy:
Physical therapy exercises can strengthen the abdominal muscles and improve overall core strength. While not a standalone treatment for hernias, incorporating targeted exercises can be beneficial in

certain cases, especially during the preoperative and postoperative phases.

The choice between surgical and nonsurgical approaches depends on factors such as the type and size of the hernia, symptoms, patient health, and the presence of complications. Individualized treatment plans, often involving a collaborative discussion between patients and healthcare professionals, ensure the most appropriate approach for each unique case. Ultimately, the goal is to provide effective hernia management while considering the patient's wellbeing and preferences.

Pros and cons of different treatments

Surgical Approaches:

Pros:

1. Effective and Permanent Repair: Surgical procedures like herniorrhaphy and

laparoscopic repair offer a direct and often permanent solution by addressing the weakened abdominal wall and securing the herniated tissue.

2. Quick Resolution: Surgery provides a relatively swift resolution to the hernia, allowing patients to return to their normal activities faster compared to nonsurgical approaches.

3. Prevention of Complications: Surgical repair helps prevent potential complications associated with untreated or recurring hernias, such as bowel obstruction or strangulation.

Cons:

1. Surgical Risks: All surgeries carry inherent risks, including infection, bleeding, or adverse reactions to anesthesia. While these risks are generally low, they should be considered.

2. Recovery Time: The recovery period after surgery varies, and some patients may experience discomfort, limited mobility, or temporary lifestyle adjustments during this time.

3. Potential for Recurrence: Although surgical repair is designed to be permanent, there is a small risk of hernia recurrence, particularly if lifestyle factors contributing to the initial hernia development are not addressed.

NonSurgical Approaches:

Pros:

1. Conservative Management: Nonsurgical approaches, such as watchful waiting, are suitable for small, asymptomatic hernias. This approach allows patients to manage the condition without immediate intervention.

2. Less Invasive: Supportive garments and lifestyle modifications are noninvasive and generally associated with fewer immediate risks and side effects compared to surgery.

3. Options for HighRisk Patients: For individuals with certain health conditions that pose surgical risks, nonsurgical approaches may provide a viable alternative.

Cons:

1. Temporary Relief: Nonsurgical options like supportive garments offer symptomatic relief but do not address the underlying issue, and hernias may progress over time.

2. Limited Effectiveness: Lifestyle modifications and physical therapy may have limitations in treating larger or symptomatic hernias, potentially leading to the need for surgical intervention later.

3. Risk of Complications: In some cases, nonsurgical approaches may not prevent complications associated with hernias, such as bowel obstruction or strangulation.

Choosing the Right Approach:

Ultimately, the decision between surgical and nonsurgical treatments involves weighing the pros and cons in the context of individual patient factors, hernia characteristics, and the overall impact on the patient's quality of life. Collaborative discussions between patients and healthcare professionals help ensure informed decisionmaking tailored to each unique case.

Collaborative decisionmaking with healthcare professionals

Collaborative decisionmaking with healthcare professionals plays a pivotal role in the comprehensive management of hernias, ensuring that patients are active participants in choosing the most suitable treatment plan for their individual circumstances. This collaborative approach fosters a partnership between patients and healthcare providers, taking into account medical expertise, patient preferences, and the unique aspects of each hernia case.

When a patient is diagnosed with a hernia, healthcare professionals typically initiate a detailed discussion to explore treatment options. This involves explaining the nature of the hernia, potential risks and benefits associated with various treatments, and addressing the patient's concerns or preferences. Importantly, this collaborative dialogue empowers patients by providing them with a clear understanding of their condition, allowing them to make informed decisions about their healthcare journey.

Healthcare professionals consider factors such as the type and size of the hernia, the patient's overall health, lifestyle, and any existing medical conditions. Surgical options, including traditional open procedures and minimally invasive techniques like laparoscopic or roboticassisted surgery, are thoroughly discussed, highlighting the advantages and potential risks associated with each approach.

Nonsurgical options, such as watchful waiting, supportive garments, lifestyle modifications, or physical therapy, are also explored based on the specific characteristics of the hernia and the patient's preferences. The collaborative decisionmaking process extends beyond simply presenting information; it involves active engagement, allowing patients to express their concerns, ask questions, and voice their preferences.

This dialogue ensures that patients have a comprehensive understanding of the implications of different treatment choices, enabling them to actively participate in crafting a personalized treatment plan aligned with their goals and values. For instance, a patient with a small, asymptomatic hernia may opt for a watchful waiting approach, appreciating the opportunity to manage the condition without immediate surgery. On the other hand, someone with a larger or symptomatic hernia may choose a surgical intervention to address the issue more definitively.

By fostering open communication and collaboration, healthcare professionals and patients work together to navigate the complexities of hernia treatment. This shared decisionmaking model recognizes the importance of tailoring interventions to the unique needs and preferences of each patient, ultimately contributing to better outcomes and patient satisfaction. The collaborative decisionmaking process extends beyond the initial treatment choice, encompassing ongoing discussions about postoperative care, recovery expectations, and longterm considerations for hernia management. This approach establishes a foundation for trust and mutual understanding, enhancing the overall patient experience and optimizing the effectiveness of hernia care.

Chapter 4: Road to Recovery

Postsurgery expectations and care

Embarking on the road to recovery after hernia surgery involves a multifaceted approach, encompassing both physical healing and attentive postsurgery care. Understanding the expectations and following prescribed guidelines are crucial for a successful recovery journey.

PostSurgery Expectations:

1. Immediate Recovery: In the initial postsurgery period, patients may experience some discomfort, pain, or swelling around the incision site. This is a normal part of the healing process and can be managed with prescribed pain medications and proper rest.

2. Activity Restrictions: While gradual movement is encouraged to prevent stiffness, patients are generally advised to

avoid strenuous activities, heavy lifting, or intense exercises during the early recovery phase. Following these guidelines promotes proper healing and minimizes the risk of complications.

3. Dietary Adjustments: Depending on the type of hernia surgery, healthcare professionals may recommend dietary modifications. In some cases, a temporary switch to a softer or lowfiber diet might be advised to ease digestion and reduce strain on the abdominal muscles.

4. Followup Appointments: Regular followup appointments with the healthcare team are crucial for monitoring recovery progress. These visits allow healthcare professionals to assess the healing of the incision site, address any concerns, and make adjustments to the recovery plan as needed.

5. Resuming Normal Activities: As recovery progresses, patients will gradually be able

to resume normal daily activities. However, the timeline for resuming activities may vary depending on the type of surgery and individual healing rates.

PostSurgery Care:

1. Incision Site Care: Proper care of the incision site is paramount. Following healthcare professionals' instructions for cleaning and dressing the incision helps prevent infection and supports optimal healing. Patients are advised to keep the incision area dry and avoid exposing it to excessive moisture.

2. Pain Management: Managing postsurgery pain is essential for a comfortable recovery. Patients are prescribed pain medications as needed, and adhering to the recommended dosage schedule helps control pain while minimizing the risk of side effects.

3. Gradual Physical Activity: Gentle, gradual physical activity is encouraged to prevent

stiffness and promote blood circulation. Healthcare professionals may recommend specific exercises or movements that are safe for the recovery phase.

4. Healthy Nutrition: A balanced and nutritious diet aids in the healing process. Patients are advised to follow any dietary recommendations provided by healthcare professionals, ensuring they get the necessary nutrients for recovery.

5. Hydration: Staying adequately hydrated supports overall recovery. Proper hydration helps the body heal, reduces the risk of complications, and supports various bodily functions during the recovery period.

6. Monitoring for Complications: While complications after hernia surgery are rare, it's essential for patients to be vigilant and promptly report any unusual symptoms, such as increased pain, swelling, redness, or signs of infection, to their healthcare team.

The road to recovery after hernia surgery is a collaborative effort between patients and healthcare professionals. Open communication, adherence to postsurgery guidelines, and a commitment to selfcare contribute to a smoother recovery journey, allowing individuals to gradually regain their strength and resume their daily activities with confidence.

Physical therapy and rehabilitation

Physical therapy and rehabilitation are integral components of the recovery process after hernia surgery. These tailored programs are designed to enhance strength, flexibility, and overall functional capacity, ensuring a smooth return to normal activities while minimizing the risk of complications. Here's an indepth look at the importance and key aspects of physical therapy and rehabilitation for hernia patients:

Importance of Physical Therapy and Rehabilitation:

1. Strengthening Core Muscles:
   Physical therapy focuses on exercises that target the core muscles, including those of the abdomen and lower back. Strengthening these muscles is crucial for providing support to the repaired hernia site and preventing future occurrences.

2. Improving Range of Motion:
   Rehabilitation programs incorporate exercises to enhance flexibility and range of motion. This is particularly important for individuals who may experience stiffness after surgery, promoting better mobility and reducing discomfort.

3. Promoting Proper Body Mechanics:
   Physical therapists guide patients in adopting proper body mechanics during daily activities. This helps prevent unnecessary strain on the abdominal

muscles, reducing the risk of hernia recurrence and supporting longterm wellbeing.

4. Addressing Scar Tissue:
   Surgical procedures can result in scar tissue formation. Physical therapy techniques, such as massage and stretching exercises, aim to minimize scar tissue restrictions and improve tissue pliability for optimal healing.

5. Pain Management:
   Physical therapists work with patients to manage any residual pain or discomfort through targeted exercises and interventions. This collaborative approach helps individuals gradually reduce reliance on pain medications.

6. Functional Rehabilitation:
   Rehabilitation programs are tailored to each patient's specific needs and goals. Whether the individual has undergone open surgery or minimally invasive procedures,

the rehabilitation plan considers the unique aspects of the hernia repair and the patient's overall health.

Key Aspects of Physical Therapy and Rehabilitation:

1. Early Mobilization:
   Initiating gentle exercises and movements shortly after surgery promotes early mobilization and prevents complications associated with prolonged bed rest. Physical therapists guide patients through safe and gradual activities based on their recovery status.

2. Progressive Exercise Program:
   Rehabilitation involves a progressive exercise program that gradually increases in intensity as the patient's strength and endurance improve. This helps individuals regain functional capacity while minimizing the risk of overexertion.

3. Education and Guidance:

Physical therapists provide education on proper body mechanics, lifting techniques, and strategies to prevent activities that could strain the abdominal muscles. This knowledge empowers patients to make informed decisions in their daily lives to protect their hernia repair.

4. Monitoring and Adjustments:
Regular monitoring of progress allows physical therapists to make necessary adjustments to the rehabilitation plan. This ensures that the program remains aligned with the patient's evolving needs and recovery milestones.

5. Home Exercise Programs:
To complement inoffice sessions, physical therapists often prescribe home exercise programs. These exercises are tailored to the individual's capabilities and provide a consistent approach to rehabilitation between scheduled sessions.

Physical therapy and rehabilitation are collaborative efforts between patients and healthcare professionals. By actively participating in these programs, individuals undergoing hernia surgery can optimize their recovery, regain physical function, and cultivate habits that contribute to longterm wellbeing. The tailored and patientcentered nature of physical therapy ensures that individuals receive the support they need throughout the entire rehabilitation journey.

Emotional wellbeing during the recovery process

Emotional wellbeing during the recovery process from hernia surgery is a crucial aspect often overlooked but profoundly impactful on the overall healing journey. Surgery, even for common procedures like hernia repair, can evoke a range of emotions, including anxiety, fear, frustration, and even relief. Understanding and addressing these emotional aspects is integral to fostering a positive recovery experience.

Patients may experience anxiety before surgery, stemming from concerns about the procedure, potential complications, or uncertainty about the outcome. Open and transparent communication with healthcare professionals can help alleviate these concerns. Presurgery counseling or educational sessions can provide a clearer understanding of the procedure, expected outcomes, and the postsurgery recovery process, offering patients a sense of control and empowerment.

The immediate postsurgery period can bring about a mix of emotions, including relief that the procedure is over and anticipation about the recovery ahead. However, patients may also grapple with discomfort, pain, or the need to depend on others for assistance during this phase. It is essential for patients to express their feelings openly to their healthcare team, who can provide support, reassurance, and guidance on managing emotional wellbeing.

Pain and physical discomfort can contribute to emotional strain during recovery. Integrating pain management strategies, including medications and alternative pain relief methods, not only addresses the physical aspect but also positively influences the emotional state. Patients should communicate any unmanageable pain levels to their healthcare team promptly.

Adjusting to activity restrictions and changes in daily routines during recovery may lead to frustration or feelings of impatience. Patients may yearn to resume normal activities, and any setbacks can be emotionally challenging. Here, setting realistic expectations, acknowledging progress, and celebrating small milestones become essential. Healthcare professionals,

UNDERSTANDING AND OVERCOMING HERNIAS

including physical therapists, play a vital role in helping individuals navigate these emotional challenges by providing encouragement and emphasizing the importance of gradual recovery.

Support systems, including friends, family, and healthcare professionals, contribute significantly to emotional wellbeing. Open communication with loved ones about emotional struggles fosters a supportive environment. Engaging in activities that bring joy, relaxation, or distraction can also positively impact emotional health during recovery.

For some individuals, the impact of surgery on body image and selfesteem may contribute to emotional challenges. Scars, changes in physical appearance, or limitations in mobility may trigger feelings of selfconsciousness. Encouraging selfcompassion and seeking professional guidance, if needed, can help address these emotional concerns.

Emotional wellbeing is an ongoing consideration throughout the recovery process. As individuals progress in their recovery journey, the emotional landscape may evolve. Transitioning from a patient role to resuming normal activities can bring about a mix of emotions, including a sense of accomplishment and, for some, anxiety about potential recurrence.

In conclusion, recognizing and addressing emotional wellbeing during hernia surgery recovery is an integral part of comprehensive care. By fostering open communication, providing emotional support, and incorporating strategies to manage anxiety and frustration, healthcare professionals contribute to a holistic recovery experience. Patients, in turn, play an active role in expressing their emotions, seeking support when needed, and embracing a positive mindset as they navigate the physical and emotional intricacies of hernia surgery recovery.

Chapter 5: Lifestyle Considerations

Dietary adjustments for better abdominal health

Dietary adjustments play a crucial role in promoting better abdominal health, particularly for individuals who have undergone hernia surgery or are looking to prevent hernia development. Making informed choices about what to eat can contribute to overall wellbeing, aid in recovery, and reduce the risk of complications. Here's an indepth exploration of dietary considerations for better abdominal health:

1. FiberRich Foods:
   Incorporating fiberrich foods into the diet supports digestive health and helps prevent constipation. Whole grains, fruits, vegetables, and legumes are excellent sources of fiber. Adequate fiber intake promotes regular bowel movements,

reducing strain on the abdominal muscles and decreasing the risk of hernia development or exacerbation.

2. Hydration:
  Staying wellhydrated is essential for maintaining healthy digestion and preventing constipation. Proper hydration also contributes to tissue healing and supports overall wellbeing. Individuals should aim to drink an adequate amount of water daily, and this can be complemented by consuming hydrating foods such as waterrich fruits and vegetables.

3. Lean Proteins:
  Including lean sources of protein in the diet is vital for muscle repair and overall recovery, especially after hernia surgery. Lean meats, poultry, fish, tofu, legumes, and lowfat dairy products are excellent protein choices. Protein supports the healing process, aids in maintaining muscle integrity, and contributes to overall strength.

4. Small, Frequent Meals:

   Opting for smaller, more frequent meals instead of large, heavy meals can help manage abdominal pressure. This approach minimizes the strain on the abdominal muscles during digestion, reducing the likelihood of discomfort or potential herniarelated complications.

5. Limiting Processed and HighFat Foods:

   Foods high in processed sugars and saturated fats can contribute to weight gain and may strain the abdominal muscles. Limiting the intake of processed foods, fried items, and sugary snacks supports overall health and helps manage body weight.

6. Avoiding Trigger Foods:

   Individuals may identify specific foods that trigger digestive discomfort or acid reflux. For those with hiatal hernias, avoiding acidic or spicy foods can help manage symptoms. Customizing the diet based on personal triggers supports digestive comfort and minimizes potential irritants.

7. Vitamins and Minerals:
  Ensuring an adequate intake of essential vitamins and minerals is crucial for overall health and healing. Foods rich in vitamin C, vitamin A, zinc, and other nutrients contribute to tissue repair and immune function. A wellbalanced diet with a variety of fruits, vegetables, whole grains, and lean proteins helps meet these nutritional needs.

8. PostSurgery Guidelines:
  Following any specific dietary guidelines provided by healthcare professionals postsurgery is essential. This may include recommendations on dietary restrictions, gradually reintroducing certain foods, or adjusting the diet to support the recovery process.

9. Mindful Eating:

Practicing mindful eating involves paying attention to hunger and fullness cues, chewing food thoroughly, and savoring the eating experience. Mindful eating can prevent overeating, reduce the risk of indigestion, and promote overall digestive health.

10. Individualized Approach:
It's crucial to recognize that dietary needs vary among individuals. Factors such as age, underlying health conditions, and personal preferences influence dietary choices. Consulting with healthcare professionals or a registered dietitian can provide personalized guidance based on individual circumstances.

In conclusion, adopting a balanced and thoughtful approach to dietary choices contributes significantly to better abdominal health. Whether recovering from hernia surgery or aiming to prevent hernia development, individuals can enhance their wellbeing by making informed dietary adjustments that support digestive health, promote healing, and contribute to overall abdominal strength.

Exercise recommendations for prevention and recovery

Exercise is a crucial component for both the prevention and recovery of hernias. Targeted exercises can strengthen the core muscles, improve flexibility, and contribute to overall abdominal health. Here's an indepth exploration of exercise recommendations for hernia prevention and recovery:

Prevention:

1. CoreStrengthening Exercises:
   Engaging in exercises that specifically target the core muscles, including the rectus abdominis, obliques, and transverse abdominis, is essential for preventing

hernias. Planks, bridges, and abdominal crunches performed with proper form can help strengthen these muscles.

2. Pelvic Floor Exercises:
   Strengthening the pelvic floor muscles is beneficial for overall abdominal support. Kegel exercises, which involve contracting and relaxing the pelvic floor muscles, can help enhance muscle tone and stability in the pelvic region.

3. Cardiovascular Exercise:
   Maintaining cardiovascular health is important for overall wellbeing and weight management. Engaging in regular aerobic exercises such as walking, jogging, swimming, or cycling can contribute to weight control and reduce the risk of obesityrelated hernias.

4. Proper Lifting Techniques:
   Learning and practicing proper lifting techniques is crucial for preventing hernias, especially in individuals whose activities

involve lifting heavy objects. Techniques such as bending at the knees, keeping the back straight, and using the legs for lifting can help reduce strain on the abdominal muscles.

5. Posture Improvement:
   Poor posture can contribute to abdominal strain. Exercises that focus on improving posture, such as shoulder blade squeezes and neck stretches, contribute to better spinal alignment and reduce the risk of developing hernias.

Recovery:

1. Gradual Resumption of Activity:
   After hernia surgery, it's important to start with gentle, lowimpact activities and gradually increase intensity. Walking and gentle stretching can be initial exercises to promote blood circulation and prevent stiffness.

2. Core Rehabilitation Exercises:

Physical therapy often includes specific exercises for core rehabilitation posthernia surgery. These exercises are tailored to the individual's recovery status and may involve movements to strengthen the repaired abdominal wall gradually.

3. Pelvic Floor Exercises:

Pelvic floor exercises continue to be relevant during the recovery phase. These exercises help restore strength to the pelvic region, contributing to overall abdominal stability.

4. Aerobic Exercise:

As recovery progresses, incorporating lowimpact aerobic exercises, such as stationary biking or swimming, can enhance cardiovascular health without putting excessive strain on the healing abdominal muscles.

5. Customized Exercise Plans:

Healthcare professionals, including physical therapists, play a crucial role in developing customized exercise plans based on the individual's specific hernia type, surgical approach, and overall health. These plans evolve throughout the recovery process.

6. Avoiding HighIntensity Workouts:
   During the initial phases of recovery, it's advisable to avoid highintensity workouts or exercises that excessively engage the abdominal muscles. Straining the healing tissues can impede recovery and increase the risk of complications.

7. Mindful Movement Practices:
   Mindful movement practices, such as yoga or tai chi, can be beneficial for both physical and mental wellbeing during hernia recovery. These practices emphasize gentle, controlled movements that promote flexibility and relaxation.

8. Regular Monitoring and Adjustments:
   Regular followup with healthcare professionals allows for monitoring of

recovery progress and adjustments to the exercise plan as needed. This ensures that the exercises align with the individual's healing trajectory and prevent potential setbacks.

In summary, a combination of targeted exercises for prevention and a gradual, tailored approach to exercise during recovery contribute to better abdominal health. The key is to prioritize proper form, listen to the body's cues, and work collaboratively with healthcare professionals to ensure a safe and effective exercise regimen tailored to individual needs and circumstances.

Two important exercises

 1. Planks for Core Strengthening:
Steps:

1. Starting Position:
   Begin by positioning yourself face down on a mat or a comfortable surface. Place

your forearms on the ground, with your elbows directly beneath your shoulders.

2. Alignment:
   Ensure that your body forms a straight line from your head to your heels. Engage your core muscles by pulling your navel toward your spine. Keep your shoulders away from your ears to avoid tension in the neck.

3. Forearm and Elbow Position:
   Plant your forearms firmly on the ground, parallel to each other. Elbows should be directly beneath your shoulders, creating a 90degree angle.

4. Leg Position:
   Extend your legs straight out behind you, balancing on your toes. Feet should be hipwidth apart. Maintain a neutral spine, avoiding any sagging or arching.

5. Hold and Breathe:

Hold the plank position for as long as you can maintain proper form. Focus on controlled breathing—inhale deeply through your nose, exhale slowly through your mouth.

6. Modifications:

For beginners, you can modify by balancing on your knees instead of your toes. Gradually progress to the full plank position as your core strength improves.

2. Kegel Exercises for Pelvic Floor Strengthening:
Steps:

1. Finding the Right Muscles:

Identify your pelvic floor muscles by imagining you're trying to stop the flow of urine or prevent passing gas. These are the muscles you'll be targeting.

2. Initial Position:

Sit or lie down comfortably. Ensure your abdominal, buttock, and thigh muscles are relaxed.

3. Isolation of Muscles:
   Tighten your pelvic floor muscles by contracting them for a few seconds. Focus on lifting and squeezing, without holding your breath or tightening other muscle groups.

4. Release and Relax:
   Relax your pelvic floor muscles completely after the contraction. Allow a complete release of tension before repeating the exercise.

5. Repetition and Progression:
   Start with a few repetitions, gradually increasing as your muscles become accustomed. Aim for a consistent routine, incorporating Kegel exercises into your daily activities.

6. Consistency is Key:

Consistency is crucial for the effectiveness of Kegel exercises. Aim to incorporate them into your daily routine, performing multiple sets throughout the day.

These two exercises, planks and Kegel exercises, target different areas of the core and pelvic floor muscles, respectively. Incorporating them into your regular exercise routine can contribute significantly to core strength, stability, and overall abdominal health. Remember to start at a level that matches your current fitness and gradually progress to more challenging variations as you build strength. If you have undergone hernia surgery or have specific health concerns, consult with your healthcare professional before starting any new exercise regimen.

Stress management and its impact on hernias

Stress management plays a notable role in overall health, and its impact extends to conditions like hernias. Stress can affect the body in various ways, potentially influencing the development, progression, or exacerbation of hernias. Understanding this connection emphasizes the importance of adopting effective stress management strategies. Here's an exploration of stress management and its impact on hernias:

1. Muscle Tension and Strain:
   Stress often manifests physically as muscle tension. Persistent tension, especially in the abdominal muscles, can contribute to increased intraabdominal pressure. This elevated pressure may strain weakened areas in the abdominal wall, potentially contributing to hernia development or aggravation.

2. Impact on Digestive Function:

Chronic stress can disrupt normal digestive processes. Conditions like irritable bowel syndrome (IBS) or acid reflux, which are associated with stress, may indirectly contribute to increased abdominal pressure. This heightened pressure can potentially contribute to the formation or worsening of hernias.

3. Immune System Function:
Prolonged stress can negatively impact the immune system. A weakened immune response may compromise the body's ability to repair tissues effectively, including the weakened areas in the abdominal wall where hernias can occur. This could potentially influence the healing process after hernia surgery.

4. Lifestyle Factors:
Stress often contributes to unhealthy lifestyle habits, such as poor dietary choices, inadequate sleep, or reduced physical activity. These factors can indirectly impact abdominal health and

contribute to conditions that may increase the risk of hernias.

5. Coughing and Straining:
   Stressrelated coughing or habitual throat clearing may increase intraabdominal pressure. Consistent straining can potentially contribute to the development of hernias, especially in individuals with preexisting weaknesses in the abdominal wall.

Effective Stress Management Strategies:

1. Mindfulness and Relaxation Techniques:
   Engaging in mindfulness practices, such as meditation, deep breathing, or progressive muscle relaxation, can help alleviate stress and reduce muscle tension. These techniques promote relaxation throughout the body, including the abdominal muscles.

2. Regular Physical Activity:

Incorporating regular exercise into your routine is a powerful stress management tool. Physical activity not only directly reduces stress but also promotes overall health, contributing to better resilience against the impact of stress on abdominal health.

3. Healthy Lifestyle Choices:
Adopting a wellbalanced diet, ensuring adequate sleep, and minimizing the consumption of stimulants (like caffeine and nicotine) can positively influence stress levels and overall wellbeing.

4. Support Systems:
Building and maintaining strong social connections can provide emotional support during stressful times. Sharing concerns and seeking help can alleviate emotional burdens that may contribute to physical tension.

5. Professional Guidance:

Seeking guidance from mental health professionals, such as psychologists or counselors, can be beneficial in developing effective stress management strategies tailored to individual needs.

Conclusion:
Stress management is a holistic approach that encompasses physical, emotional, and lifestyle considerations. While stress alone may not directly cause hernias, its impact on muscle tension, digestive function, and overall wellbeing underscores the need for effective stress management. By adopting healthy coping mechanisms and lifestyle choices, individuals can contribute to their overall abdominal health and potentially reduce the risk of hernias or complications related to hernias. If you have concerns about stress and its impact on your health, consult with healthcare professionals or mental health experts for personalized guidance and support.

Chapter 6: Prevention Strategies

Identifying and addressing risk factors

Identifying and addressing risk factors is crucial for preventing and managing hernias effectively. Understanding the factors that contribute to hernia development allows individuals and healthcare professionals to implement targeted strategies for risk reduction. Here's an indepth exploration of common risk factors associated with hernias and how to address them:

1. Age and Gender:
   Identification: Hernias can occur at any age, but they are more common in older individuals. Men are generally more prone to hernias than women.
   Addressing: Regular health checkups and awareness of potential symptoms become increasingly important as individuals age. Maintaining a healthy lifestyle and engaging in targeted exercises to strengthen the

abdominal muscles can mitigate agerelated risk factors.

2. Genetic Predisposition:

Identification: Family history can influence hernia susceptibility. If close relatives have experienced hernias, there may be a genetic predisposition.

Addressing: While genetic factors are nonmodifiable, understanding the family history allows for proactive measures. Individuals with a family history may benefit from regular checkups and lifestyle adjustments to reduce modifiable risk factors.

3. Obesity and Excess Weight:

Identification: Excess weight puts added strain on the abdominal muscles, increasing the risk of hernias.

Addressing: Weight management through a balanced diet and regular exercise is key. Achieving and maintaining a healthy weight reduces abdominal pressure and lowers the risk of hernia development.

4. Chronic Constipation and Straining:

Identification: Regularly straining during bowel movements can contribute to hernia development, particularly in the abdominal wall.

Addressing: Adequate fiber intake, hydration, and lifestyle adjustments can prevent constipation. Establishing healthy bowel habits reduces the need for straining and minimizes the risk of hernias.

5. Chronic Coughing:

Identification: Persistent coughing, often associated with conditions like smoking or respiratory issues, can contribute to hernias.

Addressing: Addressing the underlying cause of chronic coughing, such as smoking cessation or managing respiratory conditions, can reduce the risk. Seeking medical attention for persistent coughs is crucial.

6. Heavy Lifting and Strain:

Identification: Engaging in heavy lifting without proper techniques can strain the abdominal muscles, increasing the risk of hernias.

Addressing: Education on proper lifting techniques and using assistive devices when necessary can mitigate the risk. Implementing workplace safety measures is crucial for individuals with physically demanding jobs.

7. Pregnancy and Childbirth:
Identification: Pregnancy can weaken abdominal muscles, and childbirth can contribute to hernia development.

Addressing: Prenatal exercises and postpartum rehabilitation focused on core strength can help prevent and manage hernias. Consultation with healthcare professionals for personalized guidance is essential.

8. Previous Hernia Surgery:
Identification: Individuals who have undergone hernia surgery are at risk of

recurrence or developing hernias in other areas.

Addressing: Adhering to postsurgery guidelines, engaging in rehabilitation exercises, and maintaining a healthy lifestyle contribute to preventing recurrence.

9. Connective Tissue Disorders:

Identification: Certain connective tissue disorders may increase susceptibility to hernias.

Addressing: Management of underlying medical conditions and close collaboration with healthcare professionals is essential for individuals with connective tissue disorders.

Conclusion:

Identifying and addressing risk factors for hernias involve a proactive approach that combines awareness, lifestyle modifications, and, in some cases, medical interventions. By understanding individual risk profiles and implementing targeted strategies, individuals can significantly reduce the likelihood of hernia development or recurrence. Regular communication with healthcare professionals for personalized guidance ensures a comprehensive and tailored approach to hernia prevention and management.

Lifestyle changes for hernia prevention

Adopting certain lifestyle changes is instrumental in preventing hernias and promoting overall abdominal health. These modifications aim to reduce risk factors associated with hernia development. Here's a comprehensive exploration of lifestyle changes for hernia prevention:

1. Maintain a Healthy Weight:
   Explanation: Excess weight contributes to increased intraabdominal pressure, putting

strain on the abdominal muscles and potentially leading to hernias.

Lifestyle Change: Embrace a balanced and nutritious diet along with regular physical activity to achieve and maintain a healthy weight.

2. Engage in Regular Exercise:

Explanation: Regular exercise strengthens the core muscles, providing better support to the abdominal wall and reducing the risk of hernias.

Lifestyle Change: Include exercises that target the core, such as planks, bridges, and abdominal crunches, in your routine. Aim for a combination of aerobic and strengthtraining exercises.

3. Practice Proper Lifting Techniques:

Explanation: Incorrect lifting techniques can strain the abdominal muscles and increase the risk of hernias, especially in jobs that involve heavy lifting.

Lifestyle Change: Learn and consistently practice proper lifting techniques, including bending at the knees, keeping the back straight, and using the legs to lift.

4. Address Chronic Constipation:
    Explanation: Straining during bowel movements can contribute to hernia development, especially in the abdominal wall.
    Lifestyle Change: Ensure an adequate intake of fiber, stay hydrated, and establish regular bowel habits. If constipation persists, consult with healthcare professionals for appropriate management.

5. Quit Smoking:
    Explanation: Smoking can contribute to chronic coughing, which increases intraabdominal pressure and may lead to hernias.
    Lifestyle Change: Quit smoking to reduce the risk of chronic coughing and improve overall respiratory health.

6. Manage Chronic Coughing and Respiratory Conditions:

Explanation: Persistent coughing strains the abdominal muscles and can contribute to hernias.

Lifestyle Change: Seek medical attention for chronic coughing, and follow prescribed treatments for respiratory conditions. Addressing the underlying cause reduces the risk of hernia development.

7. Practice Mindful Eating:

Explanation: Overeating can lead to increased abdominal pressure, potentially contributing to hernias.

Lifestyle Change: Adopt mindful eating practices, paying attention to portion sizes and recognizing satiety cues. This can promote healthy digestion and prevent overexertion of abdominal muscles.

8. Strengthen Pelvic Floor Muscles:

Explanation: Weak pelvic floor muscles may contribute to hernias, especially in the groin area.

Lifestyle Change: Include pelvic floor exercises (Kegels) in your routine to strengthen the muscles in the pelvic region.

9. Manage Stress:

Explanation: Chronic stress can lead to muscle tension, affecting the abdominal muscles and potentially contributing to hernia development.

Lifestyle Change: Engage in stressmanagement techniques such as meditation, deep breathing, or regular physical activity to promote relaxation and reduce tension.

10. Consider Supportive Garments:

Explanation: Supportive garments, such as abdominal binders or belts, may provide additional support to the abdominal muscles, especially during activities that involve increased abdominal pressure.

Lifestyle Change: Depending on individual needs and circumstances, consider using supportive garments under the guidance of healthcare professionals.

Conclusion:

Incorporating these lifestyle changes into your daily routine can significantly reduce the risk of hernia development. It's essential to approach hernia prevention comprehensively, considering factors such as weight management, exercise, proper lifting techniques, and overall abdominal health. If you have specific health concerns or risk factors, consult with healthcare professionals for personalized advice and guidance.

Regular health checkups and early intervention

Regular health checkups and early intervention play a pivotal role in managing and preventing various health conditions, including hernias. Here's an exploration of the importance of regular checkups and early intervention for herniarelated concerns:

1. Early Detection of Hernias:
   Importance: Regular health checkups facilitate the early detection of hernias or potential risk factors. Early identification allows for timely intervention and prevents complications associated with advanced hernias.
   Action: During routine checkups, healthcare professionals can perform physical examinations, inquire about symptoms, and assess risk factors. Imaging studies may be recommended if there are concerns about hernias.

2. Monitoring Existing Hernias:
   Importance: For individuals with known hernias, regular checkups enable healthcare professionals to monitor the condition's progress, assess any changes, and provide appropriate guidance for management or intervention.

Action: Scheduled followup appointments allow healthcare providers to evaluate the hernia's size, symptoms, and impact on daily life. Adjustments to the treatment plan or recommendations for surgical intervention can be made based on the monitoring.

3. Risk Factor Assessment:
Importance: Identifying and addressing risk factors for hernias is crucial for prevention. Regular health checkups provide an opportunity to assess factors such as weight, lifestyle habits, and familial predisposition to hernias.

Action: Healthcare professionals can discuss lifestyle changes, offer guidance on preventive measures, and provide tailored recommendations based on individual risk profiles.

4. Early Intervention for Symptoms:
Importance: Early recognition of symptoms associated with hernias, such as pain, bulging, or discomfort, allows for

prompt intervention and prevents potential complications.

Action: Individuals experiencing symptoms should promptly report them during health checkups. Healthcare professionals can conduct further evaluations, recommend imaging studies, and determine the appropriate course of action, whether it's conservative management or surgical intervention.

5. Lifestyle Modification Guidance:

Importance: Regular health checkups offer an opportunity for healthcare professionals to provide guidance on lifestyle modifications that can contribute to hernia prevention, such as weight management, proper lifting techniques, and exercise routines.

Action: Through discussions during checkups, healthcare providers can educate individuals on adopting healthier habits and making lifestyle changes to reduce the risk of hernias.

6. Coordination of Care:

Importance: For individuals with hernias, regular checkups facilitate coordination between healthcare professionals, ensuring a comprehensive approach to care. This includes collaboration between primary care providers, surgeons, and other specialists if needed.

Action: Coordinated care ensures that all aspects of the individual's health are considered, leading to more effective and personalized interventions.

7. Patient Education:

Importance: Regular checkups provide opportunities for patient education, ensuring that individuals are informed about herniarelated topics, preventive measures, and the importance of early intervention.

Action: Healthcare providers can address questions, provide educational materials, and engage in open communication to empower individuals to actively participate in their hernia prevention and management.

Conclusion:
Regular health checkups serve as a cornerstone for hernia prevention and early intervention. Through proactive assessment, monitoring, and collaboration with healthcare professionals, individuals can take steps to reduce the impact of hernias on their health. Early detection and timely intervention contribute to better outcomes and an improved quality of life for individuals at risk of or dealing with hernias.

Chapter 7: Patient Empowerment

Building a supportive healthcare team

Patient empowerment is a crucial aspect of healthcare that involves actively involving individuals in their own care, decisionmaking processes, and overall wellbeing. Building a supportive healthcare team is a key component of empowering patients. Here's an exploration of patient empowerment and the role of a supportive healthcare team:

1. Establishing Open Communication:
   Patient Empowerment: Open communication between healthcare providers and patients fosters trust and ensures that individuals are well informed about their health status, treatment options, and potential challenges.
   Supportive Healthcare Team: A supportive healthcare team values transparent communication, actively listens

to patients' concerns, and encourages individuals to express their preferences and goals.

2. Collaborative Decision Making:
    Patient Empowerment: Involving patients in the decision making process regarding their care empowers them to make informed choices that align with their values and preferences.
    Supportive Healthcare Team: A collaborative healthcare team actively engages patients in decision making, explains treatment options, and considers individual preferences, fostering a sense of ownership and partnership in the care plan.

3. Providing Education and Information:
    Patient Empowerment: Knowledge is empowering. Educating patients about their health conditions, treatment options, and self care strategies enables them to actively participate in their care and make informed decisions.

Supportive Healthcare Team: A supportive healthcare team prioritizes patient education, providing clear and accessible information. This includes discussing diagnoses, explaining procedures, and offering resources that empower patients to take control of their health.

4. Recognizing Individual Goals and Preferences:

Patient Empowerment: Understanding and respecting the unique goals and preferences of each patient contributes to a sense of autonomy and empowerment.

Supportive Healthcare Team: A responsive healthcare team takes the time to understand individual patient goals, preferences, and cultural considerations. This personalized approach enhances the patient experience and strengthens the patient provider relationship.

5. Encouraging Self Advocacy:

Patient Empowerment: Empowered patients feel confident in advocating for their needs and expressing concerns. This self advocacy is a crucial aspect of navigating the healthcare system.

Supportive Healthcare Team: A supportive healthcare team encourages and supports patients in advocating for themselves. This may include providing guidance on asking questions, seeking clarification, and expressing preferences during healthcare interactions.

6. Fostering Emotional Support:

Patient Empowerment: Acknowledging the emotional aspects of healthcare and providing support for mental well being is essential for patient empowerment.

Supportive Healthcare Team: A compassionate healthcare team recognizes the emotional impact of health challenges and offers resources or referrals for emotional support. This may involve collaboration with mental health professionals or support groups.

7. Seamless Coordination of Care:

Patient Empowerment: An integrated and coordinated approach to care ensures that patients receive comprehensive and streamlined healthcare services.

Supportive Healthcare Team: A well coordinated healthcare team collaborates effectively, sharing information and ensuring that patients have a clear understanding of their care plan. This coordination reduces confusion and empowers patients to navigate their healthcare journey more effectively.

8. Respect for Diverse Perspectives:

Patient Empowerment: Recognizing and respecting the diversity of patients, including cultural backgrounds, beliefs, and values, contributes to an inclusive and empowering healthcare experience.

Supportive Healthcare Team: A culturally competent healthcare team values diversity and strives to provide patientcentered care that respects individual perspectives. This approach enhances trust and promotes patient engagement.

Conclusion:
Building a supportive healthcare team is integral to patient empowerment. By fostering open communication, collaborative decision making, providing education, recognizing individual goals, encouraging self advocacy, offering emotional support, coordinating care seamlessly, and respecting diverse perspectives, healthcare teams can create an environment where patients feel empowered, valued, and actively engaged in their health and wel lbeing. Patient empowerment leads to improved outcomes, increased satisfaction, and a more positive healthcare experience.

Advocating for oneself in the healthcare journey

Advocating for oneself in the healthcare journey is a fundamental aspect of ensuring personalized, effective, and patient centered care. Navigating the complexities of the healthcare system can be challenging, but active selfadvocacy empowers individuals to communicate their needs, make informed decisions, and collaborate with healthcare professionals. Here are essential strategies for effective selfadvocacy:

Informed Communication:
Engage in open and honest conversations with healthcare providers. Clearly express your symptoms, concerns, and preferences. Actively participate in discussions about diagnoses, treatment options, and potential risks.

Educate Yourself:
Take the initiative to learn about your health condition, prescribed medications, and recommended treatments. Being informed enables you to ask relevant questions, understand the rationale behind

decisions, and actively contribute to your care plan.

Ask Questions:
Do not hesitate to ask questions when clarification is needed. Seek explanations about procedures, test results, and potential side effects of treatments. Wellinformed questions empower you to make decisions aligned with your values and preferences.

Express Preferences and Goals:
Communicate your personal goals and preferences regarding your healthcare journey. This includes discussing factors like quality of life, treatment outcomes, and the importance of shared decisionmaking. Your input is crucial in tailoring care to your individual needs.

Seek Second Opinions:
If faced with a complex diagnosis or treatment plan, consider seeking a second opinion from another qualified healthcare

professional. This can provide additional perspectives, enhance your understanding, and contribute to more informed decision making.

Maintain Medical Records:
Keep organized records of your medical history, including test results, diagnoses, and treatments. Having a comprehensive overview of your health allows you to share relevant information with different healthcare providers and ensures continuity of care.

Know Your Rights:
Be aware of your rights as a patient. Familiarize yourself with privacy laws, informed consent processes, and your right to participate in decisions about your care. Understanding these rights empowers you to advocate for yourself within the healthcare system.

Build a Support System:

Enlist the support of friends, family, or advocates who can accompany you to appointments, ask questions, and provide emotional support. Having a supportive network strengthens your ability to navigate healthcare challenges.

Clarify Financial Matters:
Discuss financial aspects of your care, including insurance coverage, potential costs, and available resources. Clear communication about financial considerations helps prevent unexpected bills and ensures that you can access necessary care without undue financial burden.

Follow Up:
Regularly follow up with healthcare providers to discuss progress, address concerns, and adjust the care plan as needed. Consistent communication fosters a collaborative relationship and ensures that your evolving needs are considered.

In summary, effective self advocacy involves active engagement, informed communication, continuous learning, and collaboration with healthcare professionals. By taking an active role in your healthcare journey, you contribute to a patient centered approach that prioritizes your well being and aligns with your individual goals and preferences.

Encouraging a proactive and informed approach

Encouraging a proactive and informed approach to healthcare empowers individuals to actively engage in their well being. By taking an assertive role in managing health, individuals can enhance their understanding, make informed decisions, and contribute to a collaborative partnership with healthcare providers.

Initiate Open Communication:

Establishing open and honest communication with healthcare professionals is paramount. Actively share your health history, symptoms, and concerns, fostering a transparent dialogue that enables personalized and effective care.

Take Ownership of Health Information:
Be proactive in gathering and maintaining your health information. Keep a record of medications, allergies, and past medical history. This comprehensive overview aids in effective communication with healthcare providers and ensures continuity of care.

Educate Yourself:
Invest time in learning about your health conditions, treatment options, and potential lifestyle modifications. This knowledge empowers you to ask pertinent questions, actively participate in decision making, and collaborate on a care plan that aligns with your preferences.

Ask Informed Questions:
During medical appointments, pose thoughtful and informed questions. Seek clarification on diagnoses, treatment plans, and potential outcomes. A proactive approach to seeking information enhances your understanding and facilitates shared decision making.

Explore Second Opinions:
In complex or significant healthcare decisions, consider seeking a second opinion. This proactive step provides additional insights, validates recommendations, and contributes to your confidence in the chosen course of action.

Advocate for Preventive Measures:
Take a preventive stance by discussing proactive measures to maintain overall health. Engage in conversations about lifestyle modifications, screenings, and vaccinations that align with preventive healthcare guidelines.

Participate in Shared DecisionMaking:
Actively engage in shared decisionmaking
with healthcare providers. Express your
values, preferences, and goals to ensure
that the care plan is a collaborative effort
that respects your individual needs.

Seek Preventive Screenings:
Embrace a proactive attitude towards
preventive screenings and health checkups.
Regular screenings can detect potential
issues early, allowing for timely
interventions and better overall health
outcomes.

Emphasize Holistic Wellbeing:
Consider a holistic approach to wellbeing
that encompasses physical, mental, and
emotional health. Proactively address
stress, prioritize selfcare, and communicate
with healthcare providers about factors that
contribute to your overall wellbeing.

Establish a Support Network:

Cultivate a support network that includes family, friends, and healthcare advocates. Having a supportive community enhances your ability to navigate healthcare decisions, ask for assistance when needed, and maintain emotional wellbeing.

In essence, a proactive and informed approach to healthcare involves ongoing engagement, continuous learning, and active collaboration with healthcare professionals. By embracing this approach, individuals can play an integral role in shaping their health journey, fostering positive outcomes, and achieving a sense of empowerment in their overall wellbeing.

Chapter 8: Q&A and Expert Insights

Addressing common concerns and questions

Q: What are the common risk factors for developing hernias, and can they be prevented?

Expert Insight: Common risk factors for hernias include age, gender, family history, obesity, heavy lifting, and chronic coughing. While some factors are non-modifiable, lifestyle changes, weight management, and proper lifting techniques can significantly reduce the risk.

Q: Can hernias go away on their own, or is surgery always necessary?

Expert Insight: Hernias do not typically resolve on their own. While small hernias may not cause immediate issues, they often require surgical intervention to prevent complications. Consultation with a healthcare professional is essential to determine the appropriate course of action.

Q: How can one recognize the symptoms of a hernia, and when should medical attention be sought?

Expert Insight: Symptoms of a hernia may include a visible bulge, pain or discomfort, and a feeling of heaviness in the affected area. Seeking medical attention is crucial when symptoms persist, worsen, or if there is sudden severe pain, as these may indicate complications that require immediate intervention.

Q: Are there specific exercises that can help prevent hernias, and how important is core strength in this regard?

Expert Insight: Core strengthening exercises, such as planks and abdominal crunches, can help prevent hernias by providing better support to the abdominal muscles. Maintaining overall core strength through targeted exercises is crucial for reducing the risk of hernia development.

Q: What are the pros and cons of surgical and nonsurgical approaches to treating hernias?

Expert Insight: Surgical intervention is often recommended for hernias to prevent complications. While surgery carries some risks, it is generally safe and effective. Nonsurgical approaches, such as watchful waiting, may be considered for certain cases, but they don't address the underlying issue and pose a risk of complications.

Q: How long does the recovery process take after hernia surgery, and what can patients expect during this period?

Expert Insight: Recovery time varies depending on factors like the type of hernia and surgical approach. Generally, patients can return to normal activities gradually, following postsurgery guidelines. Initial weeks may involve limited activity, with a gradual return to full function over several weeks or months.

Q: Can hernias recur after surgery, and what measures can be taken to prevent recurrence?

Expert Insight: Hernia recurrence is possible, especially if lifestyle factors are not addressed. Following postsurgery guidelines, engaging in rehabilitation exercises, maintaining a healthy weight, and avoiding activities that strain the abdominal muscles are essential measures to prevent recurrence.

Q: How does emotional wellbeing impact the recovery process after hernia surgery, and are there strategies to support mental health during this time?

Expert Insight: Emotional wellbeing is integral to the recovery process. Anxiety and stress can affect healing. Strategies such as mindfulness, social support, and maintaining open communication with healthcare professionals contribute to positive mental health during hernia recovery.

Q: Are there dietary adjustments that can promote better abdominal health and reduce the risk of hernias?

Expert Insight: A balanced diet rich in fiber, hydration, and nutrients supports overall abdominal health. Maintaining a healthy weight through dietary choices can reduce the risk of hernias. Individuals should consult with healthcare professionals for personalized dietary recommendations.

Q: What role does physical therapy play in hernia recovery, and when is it typically recommended?

Expert Insight: Physical therapy is often recommended during hernia recovery to facilitate gradual strengthening of the core muscles. It helps individuals regain strength, flexibility, and proper movement patterns.

The timing of physical therapy recommendations varies based on individual recovery progress and healthcare professional assessments.

Q: Are there specific exercises recommended for hernia prevention and recovery, and how important is it to consult with healthcare professionals before starting an exercise regimen?

Expert Insight: Targeted exercises, including corestrengthening and pelvic floor exercises, are beneficial for hernia prevention and recovery. Consulting with healthcare professionals is crucial to ensure that exercises are appropriate for individual health status and recovery progress, minimizing the risk of complications.

Q: How can individuals effectively manage stress during their hernia journey, and what impact does stress have on hernias?

Expert Insight: Stress management is vital, as chronic stress can contribute to muscle tension and potentially impact hernias. Strategies such as mindfulness, relaxation techniques, regular physical activity, and seeking support from mental health professionals can help individuals effectively manage stress during their hernia journey.

Q: What are some practical tips for individuals to advocate for themselves within the healthcare system during their hernia journey?

Expert Insight: Effective selfadvocacy involves proactive communication, seeking information, clarifying doubts, and actively participating in decisionmaking. Keeping organized health records, asking informed questions, and building a supportive network are practical tips for individuals to advocate for themselves within the healthcare system.

Real life success stories of overcoming hernias

Success Story 1: James's Journey to Recovery

James, a 42yearold IT professional, discovered he had an abdominal hernia during a routine checkup. Concerned about the impact on his active lifestyle, James opted for surgical intervention. Following a successful surgery and diligent adherence to postoperative guidelines, James gradually reintegrated exercise into his routine. With the support of physical therapy and a commitment to a healthier lifestyle, James not only recovered but also improved his overall wellbeing. His success story highlights the importance of proactive management and a comprehensive approach to hernia recovery.

Success Story 2: Sarah's Resilience and Rehabilitation

Sarah, a 35yearold yoga instructor and mother of two, faced challenges when she developed a hernia postchildbirth. Determined to avoid surgery if possible, Sarah worked closely with her healthcare team to explore nonsurgical options. Through targeted exercises, including yoga practices that focused on core strength, Sarah experienced significant improvement. While embracing a holistic approach to her wellbeing, Sarah not only managed her hernia without surgery but also enhanced her physical and mental resilience.

Success Story 3: Emily's Triumph Over Recurrent Hernias

Emily, a 50yearold office manager, experienced recurrent hernias despite previous surgeries. Frustrated but determined, Emily sought specialized care and engaged in thorough consultations with her healthcare team. Together, they devised a personalized plan addressing lifestyle factors, including weight management and core strengthening exercises. Through a collaborative effort, Emily successfully navigated her journey, minimizing the risk of recurrence and enjoying a renewed sense of vitality.

Success Story 4: David's Positive Post Surgery Transformation

David, a 38yearold construction worker, faced a challenging hernia diagnosis that necessitated surgery. Initially apprehensive about the recovery process, David committed to the recommended postsurgery guidelines. With the support of physical therapy, David gradually regained strength and resumed work, taking necessary precautions. His positive postsurgery transformation showcased the importance of resilience and adherence to a tailored recovery plan for individuals in physically demanding professions.

Success Story 5: Maria's Empowerment Through Lifestyle Changes

Maria, a 45yearold teacher, discovered a hernia while experiencing discomfort. Instead of immediately opting for surgery, Maria proactively embraced lifestyle changes. With guidance from healthcare professionals, she incorporated abdominal-friendly exercises, adopted a nutritious diet, and practiced stress management. Over time, Maria not only alleviated her symptoms but also discovered a newfound sense of empowerment through her active role in hernia prevention and management.

These reallife success stories illustrate the diverse paths individuals take to overcome hernias. Each journey emphasizes the importance of personalized approaches, resilience, and collaborative efforts between individuals and their healthcare teams in achieving positive outcomes.

Printed in Great Britain
by Amazon

37844059R00069